The Science-Backed Innercises Method for
Greater Resilience and Internal Coherence

SOMATIC SUPERPOWERS

Unlock Your Inner Hero & Conquer Life's Challenges

by
SANDRA LARSEN
Mental Health Advocate
Creator of the Innercises Method

SOMATIC SUPERPOWERS

Unlock Your Inner Hero & Conquer Life's Challenges

FIRST EDITION

Copyright © 2024 by Sandra Larsen

All rights reserved. Except as permitted under U.S. Copyright Act of 1976, no part of this publication may be reproduced, distributed, or transmitted in any form or by any means, or stored in a database or retrieval system, without the prior written permission of the publisher.

Printed in the United States of America

Disclaimer: While the publisher and author have used their best efforts in preparing this book, they make no representations or warranties with respect to the accuracy or completeness of the contents of this book and specifically disclaim any implied warranties or merchantability or fitness for a particular purpose. No warranty may be created or extended by sales representatives or written sales materials. The advice and strategies contained herein may not be suitable for your situation. You should consult with a professional where appropriate. Neither the publisher nor author shall be liable for any loss or profit or any other commercial damages, including but not limited to special, incidental, consequential, or other damages.

SOMATIC SUPERPOWERS

FOREWORD

By Foster Gamble

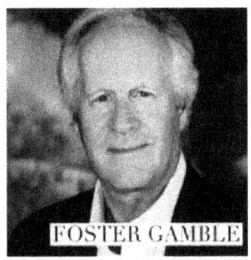

When trauma or its after-effects start to overwhelm us, what do we do first, and then what next? Does it work?

I never met a human who hasn't experienced some trauma, who doesn't need to deal with emerging stresses in their lives. There is light on this horizon. The cavalry is coming – not to do it for us, but to work with us to reclaim our joyous and true selves by learning SOMATIC SUPERPOWERS.

Our birthright is to sense when something is off, but we need to learn to identify and master the skills of dealing with turmoil effectively. These can seem like superpowers - how to recognize and clear stress and emotional blocks to restore equilibrium, joy and effectiveness. But these capabilities are not reserved for Marvel fantasy heroes with laser eyes, or fire flowing out of bladed hands. They are simple, though not necessarily easy. They are natural, yet they take deep insight and dedicated practice.

There are experts in our midst who have investigated this – who have worked hard on themselves, and ultimately became good at empowering others. Sandra Larsen is one of them.

Sandra has been working effectively with clients for many years and has distilled her findings down to this succinct and practical handbook. She hasn't spent her time collecting Hallmark platitudes or ephemeral New Age vagaries. If this seems like unfamiliar territory, you are not alone. New terms - like interoception, polyvagal, pendulation, and neuroception might seem confusing at first, but they can also be the harbingers of new relief, peace and success in your life.

Sandra is offering the best, most practical, most accessible "innercises" that she has found. This is an operating manual for troubleshooting the blockages in your life right now, and ongoingly.

She will be showing you the map and providing a compass for aligning with your body, emotions, mind and nervous system to free yourself from the freeze, fight or flight traps. You will see how to access your feelings to free your energy, to clear your mind and engage fruitfully in your best life.

I am thrilled that Sandra Larsen has taken the time to crystallize this hard-won knowledge for the rest of us and I am privileged to whole-heartedly endorse this mighty little volume. Enjoy!

- Foster Gamble, Co-creator, THRIVE Movies and Movement, Creator of LifeBalance training and former CEO of MindCenter

Contents

Introduction   1

1. Inner Space, Outer Space   5
2. First Things First   10
3. The List   14
4. HeartMath® Internal Coherence   19
5. Daily Practice   25
6. The Pause   27
7. Presence   30
8. The Butterfly Hug   33
9. Creating Awareness   35
10. Cultivate Positivity v. ANTs   40
11. The Polyvagal Theory   43
12. The Heart   47
13. Grounding   51
14. Breathwork   56
15. Meditation   59
16. Body Scan   64
17. The Five Senses   69
18. Sound   72
19. Sight   78
20. Touch   82
21. Smell   88
22. Taste   91
23. More Innercises   96

Conclusion   102
Glossary   105

"Acknowledge, accept, and honor that you deserve your own deepest compassion and love."

- NANETTE MATHEWS

Introduction

In a world constantly throwing curveballs, feeling overwhelmed, stressed, or anxious is all too common. However, with these somatic Innercises in your toolkit, you'll become inner-resourced. You will have the power to find calm amidst the chaos and build an unshakable foundation of resilience while accessing your innate super-powers.

You probably already know the importance of exercise and proper nutrition, but navigating challenging moments requires more. It requires an awareness, an acceptance, and the ability to actually DO something about it. The evidence-backed techniques in this book are designed to help you overcome any obstacle that comes your way. Each Innercise is like a hidden gem, waiting to be uncovered and polished to perfection. You will likely prefer some more than others. That is fine. As you master each one, you'll develop a greater sense of self-awareness, emotional intelligence, and courage.

The best part is that the key to unlocking your innate neural potential is already within you. You've GOT this! Are you ready to embark on a transformative journey of self-discovery and heart-centered empowerment? You can learn to unlock the secrets to experiencing inner peace, resilience to stress, and boundless potential to reach your goals and aspirations and integrate all of your abilities and goals to become the best version of yourself.

The world may offer many opportunities, but there are also limitations. This is meant to lead you toward discovering your unique power hidden within. The path emerges as you show the courage to follow your heart. You navigate your path forward with every step, breath, and thought. Without a connection to your heart, all is lost. However, having the courage to connect with your real feelings along the way can transform your path into journey 'A Hero's Journey.' Yes, you! Just like in the movie "The Never Ending Story." Do you remember it? If not, you may want to watch it again. The main character was a boy who couldn't accept that he had any power in his world. Everywhere he looked, there was chaos and trauma. The Nothingness took over, destroying the entire world and threatening the very existence of all realms. His disbelief was so strong that he refused to even try. He was in a neural state of overwhelm; "I can't." That was all he could say. The trauma he experienced left him numb and without inner connection.

At first, he became aware of the challenge, but could not accept it. Once he accepted the facts and began acting on that knowledge, Atrayu's transformation into the superhero began to take place. Once you become aware of your inner power and accept responsibility, there's no turning back. Your new path is one of transformation into the greatest version of yourself possible. Follow these practices, and you will find yourself moving rapidly toward some of the most exciting discoveries that any human has ever made. Are you ready?

Let's jump right in! We are not merely talking about it; rather, now is the time to take action. Here are a few easy steps to help you start connecting with your inner power. The more you connect with them, the more effective they become until it actually becomes second nature to you. You won't even have to think about it, and you will become inner-resourced and automatically function this way. You may ask why; what is the benefit?

The benefits are many and they are what inspired me to share this knowledge. My life has improved greatly by remembering to frequently pause and simply take a deep breath or squeeze my arms and hands as self-massage or feel into my heartbeat while remembering what I m grateful for while navigating difficult moments.

These practices help me to minimize my judgements and be more compassionate toward others. For example, a woman backed into my car in a parking lot one day. I got out and asked are you alright?" She was stunned Am I alright? I hit you!" This defused the situation, realizing that no one was injured by her mistake. She happily paid for the repairs with no animosity.

As a single parent there were times when I d just go into the bathroom and look in the mirror, breathing slowly with my hand on my heart We got this, little buddy, we got this." Remember that your heart is your little buddy, too!

Interoception: the compass that guides us through the labyrinth of our inner world.

01.

Inner Space, Outer Space

One benefit comes from expanding your ability to sense from within. Science calls this interoception. The act of sensing your inner world begins by just realizing basic things like "I feel hunger." Or "I have to go to the bathroom." Over time, with conscious effort, this can evolve into sensing other internal changes, such as "My heart is beating really fast right now." Or "My gut says not to do that." It can lead to greater presence, empathy, and intuition. You may already have a sense of this experience. Let's take it to the next level!

Interoception is the ability to be aware of internal sensations in the body, including heart rate, breathing, hunger, fullness, temperature, pain, and emotional sensations. Interoception answers the question, "How do I feel?" Can you interocept your heartbeat? How about a 'gut-feeling'? You must remind yourself at first, but it becomes second nature over time.

For example, when you walk into a room, you may get a 'feel' for it in your gut, correct? That feeling comes from sensing your environment; whether you sense it as 'safe' or 'not safe' comes from within. Your nervous system evolved this ability in order to survive. This allows for an instant response rather than taking time to think regarding life or death matters of survival.

Can you remember a time when you felt something in your gut immediately causing you to respond in such a way that later proved to be really valuable? Or maybe this happens to you all the time. Or maybe you are somewhere in between.

On a scale of zero to ten, 0——————————-10

with zero being no awareness of any inner connections or wisdom and ten being a near-constant awareness of some type of inner-connection; what number represents where you are? Does it change?

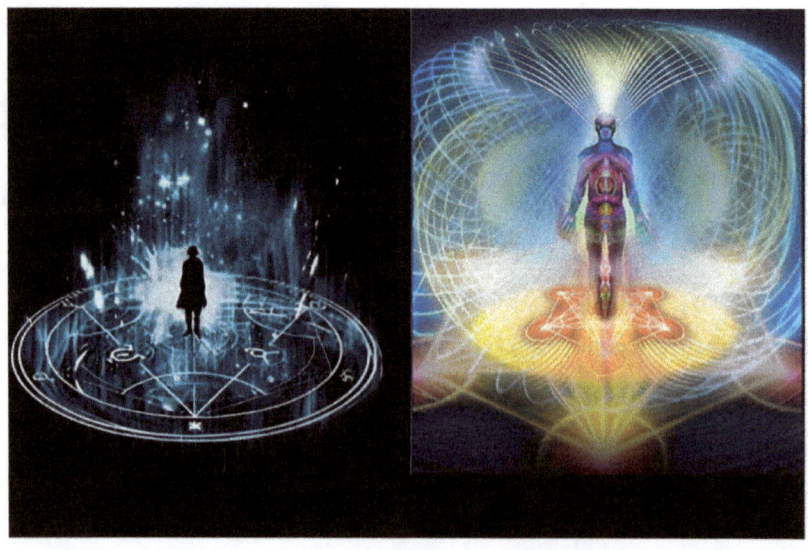

Are you at all aware of this ability and how it affects you? If not, are you willing to give it a try? Could this ability hold the key to unlocking other superpowers? Yes, it can, even those you do not know yet! You will see.

The image on the right represents our birthright: it shows the complete connection from within our inner power, radiating outward on every level. The chakras are all lit up, spinning, and vibrating in wild colors. The heart is open, and the entire electromagnetic field is radiant and rainbow-like, radiating outward. This represents an integrated human being that has evolved the capacity to impact the world and is energetically grounded to the Earth, connected above to the Light and emanating power brightly from within.

Meanwhile, the image on the left represents a human being in a state of dis-integration; there is a lack of connection from within. The world impacts them with great force. This is fear, overwhelm, and lack of power. It could be due to many things like a traumatic event leading to a freeze state of overwhelm. It could be temporary (think of a 'close call') or a long-term imprint of an intense event. It could even be an intense feeling of impending doom that just won't pass.

These two images represent the extremes of a continuum. Maybe you have experienced them both. Most of us exist somewhere between the two. Hopefully, you are heading toward the image on the right. You might not always feel so bright and shiny, but once you have experienced glimpses of it, your curiosity beckons you forth.

There are many levels to your existence. As you evolve, you learn to 'sense' into yourself, your relationships, and your environment. For some, this may be an image; for others, it may be a feeling or a thought. We each respond uniquely.

"Interoception is the ability to sense our internal state, a critical component of self-regulation. It is the process of bringing attention to the sensations, feelings, and thoughts inside our bodies. This inner awareness is essential for understanding our needs and emotions and developing the ability to regulate them effectively."

- STEPHEN PORGES

02.
First Things First

Step one is the realization of an awareness. Like a Jedi senses a disturbance in The Field. The second step is acceptance. From there, many choices emerge. So here you are, with an awareness that you would like to access and develop your inner strengths. You have accepted this as a worthy endeavor. It is okay to have doubts but keep moving forward. First things first. Remember to pause at least once every hour. Take a nice deep breath whenever you think of it. In just a couple more paragraphs, you will be ready to begin your first Innercise.

One main point to understand is that the choices you make are dependent on whether or not your nervous system is interocepting safety. The nervous system runs our physiology. For example, if you walk into a room and immediately sense that something doesn't feel right in your gut, you may choose to walk out. You will likely choose to stay if you walk into a room and feel safe.

A third possibility is that you are completely unaware of your ability to sense your environment. You may not even notice that you have happened to walk into an unsafe situation. Maybe the floor is wet and slippery, maybe someone is acting aggressively in that room, or someone sprayed poison. Not knowing can be dangerous. So critical to the survival of the human race is this knowing that you have evolved the ability to sense danger from inside your gut; this is interoception.

Remember that "Aha!" moment in 'The Never Ending Story' when Atreyu paused and realized that he does have the ability and the power from within to accept and actually respond to the threat of 'The Nothingness'? It had been so overwhelming to him, and yet his acceptance brought on the emergence of amazing superpowers beyond his wildest dreams. No longer a young, powerless child, he emerges as a superhero saving the world. What changed? It was a sense that he became aware of from within and found the courage to accept. Then he began to act. His transformation emerged from within!

When you sense safety, you have a greater capacity to feel and to interocept. You are more able to pause and connect with others. You can connect to your feelings more easily and express or process them better.

When you are not sensing safety, you tend to focus more on your thoughts about the situation and disconnect from your feelings. Thoughts can become more fearful and rapid. Maybe you've not felt safe for a period of time, and you're used to being numb. When the ability to feel, sense into, or interocept returns, your feelings may seem huge, overwhelming, or just really raw. It is important to remember that this will balance out over time as you get used to feeling again and can learn to ride the waves more gracefully. It's a process.

Interoception may not give you superpowers like flying or invisibility, but it can help you develop a kind of 'inner superpower.' By learning to tune into and understand your body's signals, you can become more aware of your emotions, make better decisions, and develop greater resilience in the face of stress and challenges. While it may not be a flashy superpower, this inner strength and self-awareness can help you navigate life's ups and downs easily and confidently.

Attending to our interoceptive signals is the key to unlocking the door between our inner and outer worlds.

03.
The List

The practice of focusing on interoceptive sensations before and after you practice an Innercise or activity is a powerfully effective strategy and can strengthen your ability to interocept. This book provides a step-by-step guide and includes a list of vocabulary words that describe possibilities regarding your current neural state and a compendium of Innercise practices to choose from.

Checking in this way can enhance your intuition and help you to awaken other superpowers. You may even surprise yourself at some point and find that you can sing really well, or you may decide to take up a new language, instrument, or hobby and find that you are really good at it. You may find that you now possess even greater talent.

This is a path toward sensing higher frequencies. You may even find gifts that you never knew you had! While it may take some diligence to practice it at first, this is a great skill set that will soon begin to take place automatically and can be profoundly life-changing.

Read over these vocabulary word lists. Note that there are four sections. Go through each section separately. As you scroll down each list of words, discover which of the words you relate to and mark down any words that 'fit' your current state:

My Thoughts are...		
Curious	Over-focused or	Hopeless
Clear mind	unfocused	Stuck
Creative	Difficult concentration	Frozen
Flexible	Negative outlook	Spacey
Focus and	Sad	Dreamy
concentration	Rigid	Confusion
Positive outlook	Repetitive thoughts	Blank
	Rapid thoughts	mind
		Forgetful

After scanning through the list of your thoughts, go to the list about feelings next, then about the body, and lastly, a list of actions. Once you complete all four sections, you will have a list of words that could describe your present neural state. Now you are ready for the next step: practice your first Innercise!

Feel free to modify your list over time and add new words if you don't see them listed here. Create your own neural vocabulary! Make it yours! While it is true that we all have the same nervous system, each of us responds uniquely. Also, your response may change over time, so take a few moments to check in every time before and after. It's a great skillset!

My Feelings Are...

Happy	Irritable	Numb
Joy	Grumpy	Apathy
Love	Annoyed	Shame
Even mood	Spiteful	
Grateful	Angry	
Confident	Rage	
Comfortable	Worried	
	Anxious	
	Afraid	
	Terror	
	Panic	

My Body Feels...

Vibrant	Tight muscles	Very tight or overly soft muscles
Relaxed muscles	Fast, shallow breath	Slow heart rate
Even breathing	Fast heart rate	Slow, shallow breathing
Moderate heart rate	Cold hands and feet	Numbness
Easy digestion and elimination	Sweaty and hot	Dizziness
Expressive facial movements	Dry mouth	Pale
Vocal prosody	Poor digestion	Unfocused eyes
	Constipation	Blurry vision
	Restless	Flat facial expression
	Agitated	Monotone voice
	Shaky	Clumsy
	Fast speech	
	Eyes darting	
	Poor sleep	

LASTLY...

My Actions with others are...

Attuned	Impatient	Disconnected
Responsive	Self-focused	Non-responsive
Interactive	Confrontational	Shut down
Patient	Avoidant	Checked out
Trusting	Defensive	Isolated
	Offended	

GREAT! Thank you for taking the time to complete this first phase of the process. This is a unique and powerful way to enhance your ability to interocept or sense within. It may take a few weeks or months to begin seeing results, but this is the path. Stay with it. Without checking into the lists before and after, it is just another activity. Adding neural connections is what makes this process so powerful, and it is brain training!

You will find a wide variety of Innercises to choose from in the following pages. You can explore them over time. Right now, just begin with this powerful yet fundamental practice from HeartMath®. Internal Coherence is a favorite! Be sure to journal about it, too. Even if you just jot down a few words, later on, you will look back, and you will be able to look back and see patterns emerge. Here we go!

Take your time with step 2. Once you complete this practice, read over the four lists again. Look for any changes. Write them down.

When we achieve internal coherence, we become the architects of our own reality, sculpting a life that resonates with our deepest truths.

04.

HeartMath® Internal Coherence

HeartMath™ Coherence is a simple yet powerful technique for self-regulation. It brings your nervous system into balance quickly by restoring coherence between your brain and your heart rhythm.

Step 1: Heart Focus

- Focus your attention on the area around your heart.
- Imagine your breath flowing in and out through your heart.
- Keep your focus there as you proceed.

Step 2: Heart Feeling

- Activate a positive or renewing feeling like appreciation, care, or love.
- Feel that emanating from your heart as you breathe.

Step 3: Heart Breathing

- Notice your breathing slowing and becoming more deep as you maintain heart focus. Feel your breath coordinate with your heartbeat.

Step 4: Maintain

- Continue heart-focused breathing for a few minutes while sustaining the positive feeling. Feel into it rather than think about or judge the feelings.

Now, please read through the lists again (below). As you scroll down through each list of words, discover which, if any of the words relate to your present state. Mark down any words that 'fit' your current state. Look for any shifts or changes. What do you notice? Has anything shifted or resolved?

The Quick Coherence® technique was developed by and is a registered trademark of HeartMath." FOUND HERE: https://www.heartmath.com/trademarks/

My Thoughts are...		
Curious	Over-focused or unfocused	Hopeless
Clear mind		Stuck
Creative	Difficult concentration	Trapped
Flexible		Frozen
Focus and concentration	Negative outlook	Scattered
	Rigid	Spacey
Positive outlook	Repetitive thoughts	Dreamy
		Confusion
	Rapid thoughts	Blank mind
		Forgetful

My Feelings Are...

Happy	Irritable	Numb
Joy	Grumpy	Apathy
Love	Annoyed	Shame
Even mood	Spiteful	Paralyzed
Grateful	Angry	Shocked
Confident	Rage	
Comfortable	Worried	
	Anxious	
	Afraid	
	Terror	
	Panic	

My Body Feels...

Vibrant	Tight muscles	Very tight or overly soft muscles
Relaxed muscles	Fast, shallow breath	Slow heart rate
Even breathing	Fast heart rate	Slow, shallow breathing
Moderate heart rate	Cold hands and feet	Numbness
Easy digestion and elimination	Sweaty and hot	Dizziness
Expressive facial movements	Dry mouth	Pale
Vocal prosody	Poor digestion	Unfocused eyes
	Constipation	Blurry vision
	Restless	Flat facial expression
	Agitated	Monotone voice
	Shaky	Clumsy
	Fast speech	
	Eyes darting	
	Poor sleep	

My Actions with others are...		
Attuned	Impatient	Disconnected
Responsive	Self-focused	Non-responsive
Interactive	Confrontational	Shut down
Patient	Avoidant	Checked out
Trusting	Defensive	Isolated
	Offended	

Congratulations! You did it! Thank you for taking the time to complete all three phases of this process. This is a unique and powerful method to enhance your ability to interocept. With practice, sensing your current neural state will become second nature, but for now, it is important to go through this process each time.

It will be an ordinary activity without checking in using the lists before and after. Creating an increase in neural connections is what helps make this process so powerful.

Take your time getting to know all of the Innercises in this book. You can choose to stay with this Internal Coherence Practice or pick another; you can even stack them and do more than one at a time if that works for you. Explore what works for you over time. Some people prefer certain practices over others.

You will find a copy of the vocabulary lists at the end of this book.

1 Prepare by checking the words in the list

2 Choose and practice the Innercise recipe

3 Review the list again, noticing any changes

"The secret to unlocking your inner strength and resilience lies in the power of a daily somatic practice – a sacred ritual that nourishes your mind, body, and soul."

-SANDRA LARSEN

05.
Daily Practice

As you progress, this three-phase practice doesn't take long at all. Initially, it's a little slower, but the more you practice, the more quickly it flows and becomes a part of your day. Soon, you won't even skip a beat; it will become more automatic, and your abilities will expand over time. Your attention and intention will become more focused. You may even become more intuitive. Give this practice time and be consistent. The more frequently you engage with these Innercises, the sooner you will see results. Celebrate even little successes.

We each have an inner world and an outer world. Some people are more connected internally than others. That is fine, but doing the work to become more connected internally can lead to a new sense of agency moving forward. This can lead you down an entirely different path than those who are not connected internally. The evolution of your Superpowers begins now!

In the sacred space between stimulus and response lies the power to pause – a transformative gift that allows us to choose our path forward with intention and grace.

06.
The Pause

Beginning each day with the intention to pause and check in before you do anything can greatly impact your progress. Explore having a daily ritual of taking ten deep breaths while feeling what you are grateful for before you begin your day. This can allow your nervous system to have a little more resilience.

Some days, you may have more time and can add to this, making it a morning ritual, for example; try a body scan, meditation practice, or self-massage. Beginning each day with a sense of safety allows for more presence and calm during your daily activities, rather than running on automatic pilot and later wondering where the day went. Some people prefer to do this in the evening due to their schedule. That's fine, either or both! Just as long as you have a daily habit of beginning your day with even a brief interoception practice.

> *FIRST THING before you get out of bed:*
>
> *Take 10 deep breaths while focusing on what you feel gratitude or love toward.*

If there are days that you do not engage in any of these practices, don't get down on yourself; just notice. Make sure you do it the next day. You can even laugh about it. "Oh my, I never once paused to check in today!" Some days are just like that. It's okay; that is just a part of being human. More importantly, celebrating the process and keeping a positive tone to your self-talk will bring results faster. The world can get a little edgy at times, so knowing that you won't beat yourself up all day with your self-talk can resolve some anxiety.

> *Watch your inner dialogue; speak kindly to yourself.*

A brief pause, with your hand on your heart, as you take a deep breath can interrupt activation into neural states of defense such as fight, flight, or freeze. You may even begin to sense your heart as your little buddy. "I got you, we got this, let's do this!" This results in a better outcome rather thn "Oh, no... I'm so dumb!"

You can kid yourself into thinking it doesn't matter, but here's a secret: it ALL matters. YOU matter. Take it slow. Enjoy every sandwich. You will make better choices and see better results.

Presence is the key that unlocks the door to the wonder and beauty of the here and now.

07.
Presence

Find yourself a quiet moment where you can go within and turn down the volume of your thoughts for a few moments.

> - Begin Humming softly or even the whisper of a hum.
> - Now place your hand on your body where the sound resonates.
> - Place your hand on top of your head and send the vibration up and out the top of your head.
> - Now place one hand on your heart and the other on your belly. Sense into that vibration and bring it back down to your heart.
> - Make a whisper-hum sound
> - Now open your mouth while making that sound.

So much can be released through those sounds. So much can be restored, too.
Do you feel more present afterward?
Sense into it and journal about any changes you notice.

There is an internal Light within you. One that you can direct using your attention and intention. This is physics, not woo-woo.

There are several different ways to hold this information. Each one is valid. You will find a way to hold it that suits you best. Play with it! As you begin to feel more safe and present, you will be more excited about making sure that you are pausing to practice an Innercise or two throughout your day.

Maybe you want to keep things scientific, which is great; take notes and journal, and over time, you will begin to see the results of your experiment. Or maybe you feel more playful and choose to evolve into a hero with superpowers. This is your choice; you can even change how you hold it, so explore. Either way, these are internal gifts that no one knows about but YOU. Have fun with this!

The Butterfly Hug: a gentle embrace that soothes the soul and mends the wounds of the past.

08.
The Butterfly Hug

1. Cross your arms over your chest, with your fingers resting just below collarbone and thumbs as if you are giving yourself a hug. Your fingers should be pointing toward your collar bones, and your thumbs hooked.

2. Start tapping your hands alternately on your shoulders as if your fingers are the wings of a butterfly. Tap at a pace that feels comfortable and soothing to you.

3. Focus on your breathing while you are tapping. Take slow, deep breaths, and try to relax your body as much as possible.

4. Visualize a calm, safe place while tapping, such as a beautiful beach or a peaceful forest.

5. Practice the Butterfly Hug regularly, even when you are not feeling stressed or anxious. This can help you become more familiar with the technique and make it easier to use when needed.

"Physical self-awareness is the first step in releasing the tyranny of the past."

- BESSEL A. VAN DER KOLK

09.
Creating Awareness

Remember that there is an awareness correlated to these activities. For example, you may feel that you have a new awareness regarding whether you are sensing safety or danger. So, when you sense that you are NOT safe, you can immediately recognize that and act accordingly until you are once again safe. Soon, you will find that you spend less time wondering whether or not you are safe; rather, you will know from learning the cues your body sends: my breathing has slowed back down, my heartbeat isn't so rapid, or I am sleeping better lately.

Now, you can use the image of becoming an ocean of safety with little islands of 'not-safe' to negotiate over time. You can learn to trust your inner voice as an inner knowing. You can trust that you will sense a 'wrinkle' or a 'disturbance in the field' if there is danger or a threat. This also adds to your sense of trusting yourself. Your entire worldview shifts toward feeling a greater sense of safety and believing in your ability to impact your world.

Without that inner awareness, you may not even have a sense of dangerous situations until it's too late. You may feel like you exist in an ocean of danger with only little islands of safety. You might constantly fear random acts of danger in your world. You may even find it more of a challenge to trust anyone or anything. You may feel negatively impacted by the world. Not knowing, in and of itself, can result in anxiety, chronic fear, and disease.

When trusting from within, you can better sense your own instincts and follow your gut feelings. This leads to greater safety and allows more time to be spent in internal coherence, where the body functions best. This is known as homeostasis, the capacity to restore balance and wholeness.

There are many ways to move forward with this knowledge. Take your time with it. Remember, it's a process. As you familiarize yourself with the practices listed in the following pages, celebrate even the smallest successes! Whether a simple pat on the back or some kind of treat, it is important to celebrate it. Remember that all feelings are valid. Diversity is our strength, so forge ahead and enjoy each phase of this process as you create your own path ahead.

The purpose of practicing internal coherence is to neurally reconnect your brain and your heart. The nervous system controls all other systems. Befriending and working with your nervous system is how superpowers are nurtured.

You will find an image at the end of this book illustrating The Polyvagal Theory (Dr. Stephen Porges). The area at the bottom shows your nervous system interocepting safety, your systems all function optimally. The middle area describes the shift when you sense danger; your inner resources are activated in order to fight off or flee the danger until you return to safety. Some of your functions can even shut down or be altered as you mobilize for an attack. The upper section is the freeze or overwhelm state. That is, "I can't" think or feel numbness and collapse when facing a threat to life.

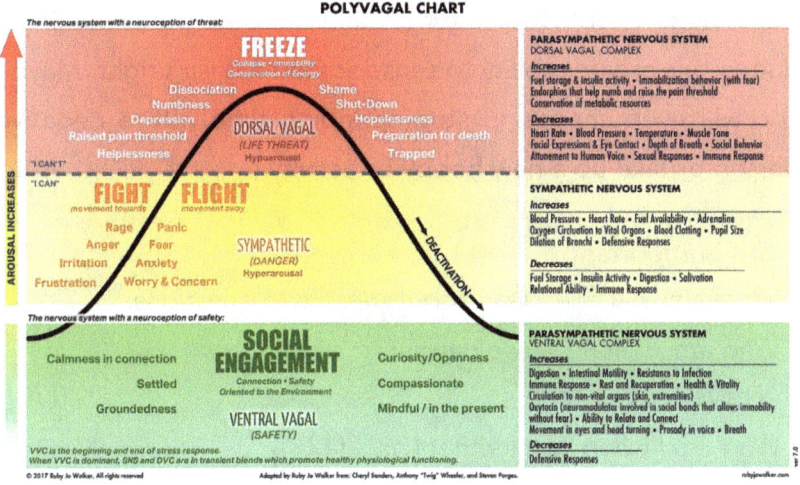

You function best when you sense safety; you can even restore balance (homeostasis) and heal most readily when in that state. Yes, the body can heal. This is where you are meant to spend most of your time, being present and connecting with others. Peace and joy. Do you notice how you are almost like two different people when you are sensing safety versus when you sense danger?

Maybe you realize that your breath becomes shallow and rapid when you sense danger. Maybe you talk faster. Maybe your muscles suddenly feel extra tense. Maybe you aren't digesting food properly or having issues with sleep. It's different for everyone. Remember, awareness is the first step. Interoception creates awareness. The next step is acceptance; you choose your best path from there.

Once you develop this greater awareness of your current state, you will begin to pause and check in automatically. You may even decide to exit a room because it doesn't feel right, turn off the television, or "Oops, I forgot that I left the water running!" due to this greater ability to sense something isn't right. Maybe you will even choose to stop spending time with a negative person or take up a new hobby or activity.

> *This is important.*
> *Write down a few ideas about these two questions:*
> *Who am I when I sense danger?*
> *"I have tended to_____."*
> *Who am I when I sense that I'm safe?*
> *"I am _____."*
> *Get to know the difference.*

- How is your inner dialogue?
- Is it kind?
- Or is it negative?
- We all face negative thoughts.

ANTs, or Automatic Negative Thoughts, are the pesky uninvited guests that buzz around our minds, clouding our judgment and stinging our self-esteem.

10.
Cultivate Positivity v. ANTs

We all face negative thoughts from time to time. These automatic negative thoughts (ANTs) are often neural remnants of an ancient survival strategy that no longer serves us in modern life. Our minds have developed a tendency to focus on negative aspects of reality to keep us safe in a world full of threats. However, in today's world, dwelling on the negative can hinder our mental health and well-being.

One effective way to combat ANTs is to counter each negative thought with three positive ones. When you catch yourself thinking negatively, simply acknowledge the thought by saying, "Cancel, cancel!" and then restate it in a positive way. Shift your focus to three positive aspects of your life or the situation at hand. By training your mind to focus on the positive, you can build resilience to ANTs and protect your mental health when life gets challenging.

Practice: *cultivate a kind inner dialogue*

> **Practice gratitude:**
> *Regularly reflect on the things you appreciate in your life, both big and small.*
>
> **Reframe challenges:**
> *Try to view obstacles as opportunities for growth and learning rather than insurmountable problems.*
>
> **Celebrate your wins:**
> *Acknowledge your accomplishments and give yourself credit for your efforts, no matter how minor they may seem.*
>
> **Be your own best friend:**
> *Talk to yourself with the same compassion, understanding, and encouragement you would offer a close friend*
>
> **Surround yourself with positivity:**
> *Seek out supportive, optimistic people who uplift and inspire you.*

Remember, experiencing negative thoughts is a normal part of the human experience. The key is to develop a healthy relationship with these thoughts and not allow them to dominate your mental landscape. Don't believe everything you think! By consistently practicing techniques like countering ANTs with positive thoughts, you can gradually reshape your inner dialogue to be more balanced, self-compassionate, and resilient.

> "Safety is the treatment."
>
> – STEPHEN PORGES PHD

11.
The Polyvagal Theory

When your nervous system gets activated into neural states of defense, including fight, flight, or freeze states, the first thing that shifts is your connection to your heart. In order to survive, you protect your heart by blocking off your feelings. You must think very clearly. You may even put those feelings into a box somewhere within your mind because they are so overwhelming. That is okay. There may be a time when you revisit it.

All feelings are valid. If you find them overwhelming, you can choose to store them away until you feel safe enough to address them or learn to hold them differently. It's that "I can't" feeling. Whatever it is, I can't deal with this right now. This is a survival tactic of the nervous system. You need to function, not go into a freeze state. Thankfully, you have that option. It takes courage to decide to store overwhelming feelings away for later. However, you need to honor your heart. You can't just pretend or deny… at least not for long. "I'm okay, I'm fine, really." It can be a trauma response rather than a fact. Denial is a strategy for some. You may find that you need help navigating those feelings; plan for that and give it a time frame to process it with a professional or a good friend.

When you sense safety, you are more comfortable negotiating your feelings. You can feel into them. Have you heard the phrase "You have to feel it in order to heal it"?.' You may also find that you make eye contact more frequently, smile more, or even reach out to connect with others more readily.

When you can create harmony and balance within yourself, it emanates outwards into your environment as a frequency. You then resonate with an external reality that exists in harmony and balance.

All living things pulsate. Life pulsates. There is an expansion phase and a contraction phase to every breath and every heartbeat. When you lose your sense of safety, the pulse contracts but doesn't fully expand, so the pulsation becomes smaller and constricted. You are alive, but maybe not so lively.

When full pulsations are restored through this work, you need to be ready for the possibility of feeling some big feelings. If you were numb or barely feeling anything for a period of time, these full pulsations may take you by surprise at first. You may have thoughts such as, "That feels so big and so raw, it might overwhelm me." But you will find it is just an adjustment period back toward your normal healthy pulse of life. Not all big feelings are overwhelming, so stay with the process if possible. Breathe through it, give yourself time, and be patient.

The heart is the guardian of our inner sanctuary, gently guiding us back to wholeness with each tender beat.

12.
The Heart

The awareness and acceptance of your feelings is the path to your strongest superpower. Many of us are connected with our hearts, but many people have chosen to protect their hearts in a way that disconnects them from their feelings. This is why it has been said, "The longest journey is from the head to the heart." Everywhere you look, you see evidence of what people think. But not so much about what they (really) feel. Their feelings are often either hidden or suppressed by things like pharmaceuticals, toxins, or fear.

In school, we learn that the heart is a pump. However, the heart is much more exciting than that. It is actually made up of seven layers of muscle that form a vortex! This vortex creates a really strong suction. So, while the heart does pump, the power of the suction from this vortex is what is so amazing. It's toroidal!

The heart's electromagnetic field can extend outward even further than that of your whole body's electromagnetic energy field. The heart even has its own nervous system. The heart's neurons mostly inform the brain; this is where saying "I had a gut feeling" comes from. We have been taught that it is the brain that thinks and the heart that feels, but it turns out that it is the heart that informs the brain.

The Heart's Electromagnetic Field

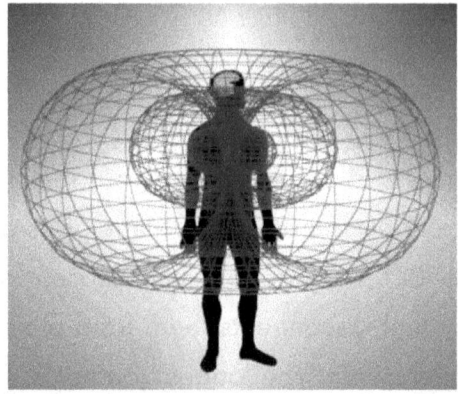

Figure 12. The heart's electromagnetic field—by far the most powerful rhythmic field produced by the human body—not only envelops every cell of the body but also extends out in all directions into the space around us. The cardiac field can be measured several feet away from the body by sensitive devices. Research conducted at IHM suggests that the heart's field is an important carrier of information.

We now understand that thoughts don't originate inside of the brain; rather, the brain is like an antenna or receiver, and thoughts actually exist in the electromagnetic field. So, don't believe everything you think! Some of those thoughts aren't even yours; you just happened to have picked them up along the way. This may help you let go of thoughts that no longer serve you. As you discover more of your inner connectedness, you become more aware of your thoughts. You can even use things like affirmations to alter repetitive thoughts.

The ability to restore internal coherence to your nervous system can lead to superpowers. Having the awareness to consciously 'pause,' feel the heart, and feel positive feelings simultaneously becomes easier and easier IF you remember to practice it! This can be a challenge if we are in an activated state, but it is easy to practice anywhere, anytime, and no one even needs to know that you are doing it. Some even use Post-it notes to remember in the beginning or tie a string around their finger or wrist. Superpower training camp!

Sometimes, when you think about doing something, an inner voice may say, "Nah, that's too difficult. Forget it." But if you push yourself, once you get going, you are so glad that you got motivated and are actually having a great time. Well, that first stage is just a phase of the motivation cycle. Some people move through that cycle more easily than others. Push yourself, but gently. Visualize success and keep moving forward.

Grounding is the gentle art of rooting ourselves in the present moment, finding stability and balance amidst life's ever-shifting tides.

13.
Grounding

A large percentage of your neurons are connected to your basic 5 senses. You use them to see, hear, taste, touch, and smell. Now, you can use this knowledge to create greater access to your Superpowers!

Once you are spending more time feeling safe, you begin to explore and expand your consciousness. One easy way involves using the 5 senses. The reason it works so well has to do with one of our nerves, the vagus nerve. Vagus means traveler, and this nerve travels to each one of our systems (digestion, circulation, etc.). The vagus nerve can instantly switch all systems into and out of activated states. It's the main switch. When this switch works properly, one is said to have a 'good vagal tone.' When it doesn't switch, it just remains in some chronic activated state (anxious, depressed, can't sleep, etc.) or gets stuck in a neural loop, and that can wear us down quickly. This known as having a lack of vagal tone.

This practice might also take a few moments at first; however, in practicing it daily, you will soon find that you can do this swiftly and without anyone even noticing AND that it works. This neural hack can help reset the nervous system out of fight, flight, or freeze back into safety.

> **IMPORTANT:**
> *Before and after this practice, please remember to scan the four lists to sense your current neural state. Interocept! That is how you create new neurons and hone new superpowers!*

Ready?

Practice: *Grounding*

> Take a nice deep breath and let it out.
>
> Now look around, even turn your head and look behind, and describe what you see.
>
> Name items or pick a color and see how many things you can find in that color.
>
> Listen; what do you hear? Describe it; which ear do you hear it out of?
>
> What can you smell? Or what are two of your favorite smells?
>
> What can you taste? Or what are two of your favorite tastes?

> Now, place your hand to touch your skin somewhere, like your arm. Describe what you feel; is it smooth or rough, wet or dry, cold or warm, etc? Is your hand sensing your arm? Is your arm sensing your hand?
>
> Now, take another deep breath.

Lastly, go back and scan the vocabulary lists again and notice what, if anything, shifted.

Take notes. Journal. Over time, you will enjoy looking back at these experiences. As you learn about your favorite things, you can use them to hack your nervous system when you sense you are becoming activated. Maybe gather some lavender or rosemary essential oil, a ginger chew or chocolate, a tuning fork or harmonica, a piece of silk or something soft or squishy, and a little love note to yourself.

Some moments are just difficult, and we just need to navigate through them. Not being able to 'DO anything about it' can feel traumatic. Having options of ways you can respond can help you to shortcut it to a better moment. Give it a try!

> *Each time you practice an INNERCISE*
> *the act of reviewing the list*
> *BEFORE and AFTER*
> *is what supports neural enhancement*
> *of your emerging superpowers.*
> *Don't skip these important steps in the process.*
> *It matters.*

Create a little sensory pouch to keep handy:

As you learn more about your favorite things, you can use them to hack your nervous system back online when you sense that you are being activated.

Find a little bag that is special to you and add to it the following:

something that you like the smell of,
something you like the taste of,
something that you like the sound of,
something you like to look at and
textures that you like the feel of.

Keep this bag with you, and when you sense that you might be getting activated, you can use it to distract your nervous system from activating and return to feeling calm and present.

"Just when the caterpillar thought the world was ending, he turned into a butterfly."

- PROVERB

14.
Breathwork

The quickest way to reconnect is through the use of your breath. Any time you remember take a nice long breath! You can even choose to release sound on the exhale…ahhhhh. Focusing on the breath can help pause the 'monkey mind' or chatter for just a second. That second can be just long enough to remind us that it's time to pause and practice Innercises.

There are many different techniques used in therapeutic breath work. They are all effective. Some more so than others. The bottom line is that each breath is sacred, and each breath has its own natural conclusion. So, use those techniques only as much as they work for you. Holding your breath can be tricky, but nice, long breaths are always good. If you feel a tightness in your ribcage, focus on expanding your belly and then your ribcage as you inhale to help unlock the diaphragm. The diaphragm is a pancake-shaped muscle at the base of the ribcage; releasing it can really make a big difference in how deeply you inhale.

Also, focus on the area below your nostrils and above your lip. Can you feel the warmth from your breath? Moisture? Can you hear your breath? What do you smell?

When practicing the Internal Coherence HeartMath® style of breathing, remember that this strategy becomes most powerful when you can *actually close your eyes and FEEL a positive feeling*. Not thinking about a feeling, but remember *feeling* that feeling in that moment; feel it again.

The root of the word heart is Latin; 'cour' refers to courage. It takes courage to feel. It's our heart that feels. When we are afraid, we really lose our ability to feel and we just numb out. The more comfortable we are regarding our feelings, the better.

"You don't have to control your thoughts. You just have to stop letting them control you."

- DAN MILLMAN

15.
Meditation

Meditation is an ancient practice that dates back thousands of years. It has gained significant popularity in recent times, especially for its remarkable effects on the nervous system. As science delves deeper into the benefits of meditation, it's becoming increasingly clear that this practice offers profound advantages for our mental and physical well-being, largely through its influence on the nervous system.

One of the most significant effects of meditation is its ability to activate the parasympathetic nervous system, promoting relaxation and reducing stress. Techniques such as deep breathing and mindfulness meditation stimulate the vagus nerve, which plays a key role in regulating the parasympathetic response.

Chronic stress can have detrimental effects on the nervous system, leading to various health issues. Meditation has been shown to lower levels of cortisol, the primary stress hormone, and reduce activity in the amygdala, the brain's center for fear and stress responses. As a result, regular meditation can help alleviate anxiety and promote a sense of calm.

Meditation has been linked to structural and functional changes in the brain, particularly in regions associated with attention, memory, and emotional regulation. Studies using neuroimaging techniques have demonstrated that meditation can increase gray matter density in areas such as the prefrontal cortex and hippocampus, which are involved in cognitive processes and emotional control.

By modulating activity in the amygdala and other emotion-related brain regions, meditation can enhance emotional resilience and reduce reactivity to negative stimuli. This can lead to improved mood regulation and a greater sense of well-being.

Meditation helps restore balance between the sympathetic and parasympathetic nervous systems, promoting overall physiological harmony. This balance is essential for optimal health, as it allows the body to efficiently respond to stressors while also conserving energy and promoting recovery.

Chronic stress weakens the immune system, making individuals more susceptible to infections and illnesses. By reducing stress and inflammation, meditation can bolster immune function and improve the body's ability to fight off pathogens.

Meditation has been shown to reduce the perception of pain by altering the way the brain processes pain signals. Techniques such as mindfulness meditation can increase pain tolerance and provide relief for chronic pain conditions.

Incorporating Meditation into Your Routine

Incorporating meditation into your daily routine can have profound effects on your nervous system and overall well-being. Here are some tips for getting started:

1. **Start Small:** Begin with just a few minutes of meditation each day and gradually increase the duration as you become more comfortable with the practice.
2. **Find a Quiet Space:** Choose a quiet, comfortable space where you won't be disturbed during your meditation sessions.
3. **Focus on Your Breath:** Pay attention to your breath as you meditate, using deep, slow breaths to anchor your awareness in the present moment.
4. **Practice Mindfulness:** Bring your attention to the present moment by focusing on your senses, thoughts, or bodily sensations without judgment.
5. **Be Consistent:** Aim to meditate regularly, even if it's just for a few minutes each day. Consistency is key to experiencing the full benefits of meditation.
6. **Experiment with Different Techniques:** Explore different meditation techniques, such as mindfulness, loving-kindness, or body scan meditation, to find what works best for you.
7. **Be Patient:** Remember that meditation is a skill that takes time to develop. Be patient with yourself and allow yourself to progress at your own pace.

In conclusion, meditation offers a powerful means of positively influencing the nervous system, promoting relaxation, reducing stress, and enhancing overall well-being. By incorporating meditation into your daily routine, you can tap into its numerous benefits and cultivate a greater sense of peace and balance in your life.

Practice: *Pre-Meditation*

- *Create a daily self-compassion ritual using phrases and activities that resonate with you.*
- *Beginning your day, this way supports a greater vagal tone over time.*
- *One example is to take 10 long breaths while feeling gratitude and love.*
- *You can add self-massage, stretching, singing, or whatever you choose on any given day.*
- *Check in on your self-talk, make sure it is positive, and practice self-compassion when you face challenges or emotional distress.*
- *By nurturing self-compassion, you promote healing and resilience in the face of past traumas—post-traumatic growth.*

The Body Scan is a sacred journey of self-discovery, illuminating the hidden landscapes within and inviting us to embrace the wholeness of our being.

16.
Body Scan

There are so many styles of meditation. The body scan is one example of how to connect in a meditative way. So, practice focusing your Laser Lightsaber attention as you scan your body. Maybe you will find it first in your heart, then bring it up to the top of your head and feel it move down your skull, over your forehead, eyes, ears, nose, and mouth, down the throat, lungs, shoulders, arms, hands, and fingers and back down through all of your organs, your spine, the pelvic bowl, down your thighs, knees, calves ankles heels and toes. Phew! Woosh!

Now try feeling it like a waterfall washing away that which no longer serves you. Or alternately, feel it upwelling from the Earth into your feet, legs, torso, etc., filling you with healing white light within and between every cell, restoring wellness and releasing that which no longer serves you.

That same practice can be used for self-healing. You can even rub your hands together to increase your energy frequency and then place your hands on an area that calls to you, like your belly, head, or heart. Play with your ability to extend your energy from within and draw it back in when you finish.

Practice: *Body Scan*

> - *Find a comfortable position while lying down with your arms at your sides and your eyes closed.*
> - *Begin at your feet and slowly scan your body, paying attention to any areas of tension, discomfort, or relaxation.*
> - *As you encounter tension, visualize it softening and melting away with each breath.*
> - *Progressively move up through your legs, torso, arms, neck, and head, continuing to observe and release any tension you find.*
> - *Conclude by focusing on your breath and the overall sensation of your body as a whole.*

The Body Scan is a powerful mindfulness practice that involves systematically focusing your attention on different parts of your body, from head to toe, with a spirit of curiosity, openness, and non-judgment. There are many variations, you can customize it to your needs. By tuning into the subtleties of physical sensation, you can cultivate a deeper sense of presence, self-awareness, and self-compassion.

The Power of the Body Scan over time:

- **Enhancing body awareness:** It helps you develop a more refined and nuanced understanding of your physical experience, allowing you to notice sensations, tensions, and areas of ease that you may have previously overlooked.
- **Promoting relaxation:** By directing your attention to each part of your body in a systematic way, the Body Scan can help you release tension, calm your nervous system, and experience a profound sense of relaxation and ease.
- **Cultivating self-compassion:** The Body Scan encourages you to approach your physical experience with kindness, gentleness, and acceptance, rather than judgment or criticism. This attitude of self-compassion can extend beyond the practice, fostering a more loving and accepting relationship with your body and yourself.
- **Integrating mind and body:** The Body Scan helps bridge the gap between your mental and physical experience, promoting a sense of wholeness and integration. By connecting with your body in this way, you can access a deeper sense of grounding, stability, and inner wisdom.

Incorporating the Body Scan into your daily routine can be a powerful way to cultivate greater self-awareness, self-compassion, and inner peace. Whether you practice for a few minutes or a full hour, the Body Scan offers a sacred space for self-discovery and self-care, inviting you to embrace the fullness of your being with each mindful breath.

Our senses are the gateways through which we experience the richness and beauty of the world around us, each one offering a unique portal into the present moment.

17.
The Five Senses

Attention and intention can play a pivotal role when working with our five senses. Just remember before each practice to clarify your intention and really pay attention to what you are doing. Scan over the lists before and after so that you can note any changes. This makes a huge difference.

The five senses – sight, sound, smell, taste, and touch – are powerful tools for cultivating mindfulness, grounding ourselves in the present moment, and savoring the fullness of our experience. By intentionally engaging with each sense, we can enhance our awareness, deepen our appreciation for the world around us, and find greater joy and peace in everyday life.

Integrating the Five Senses:

- **Mindful moments:** Choose one sense to focus on during a specific activity, such as listening intently to the sound of water as you wash dishes or savoring the aroma of your morning coffee.

- **Nature immersion:** Spend time in nature, engaging all your senses to fully appreciate the beauty and wonder of the natural world. Notice the colors of the sky, the scent of the earth, the texture of tree bark, and the sound of rustling leaves.
- **Sensory meditation:** Create a dedicated sensory experience, such as a mindful tea ceremony or a slow, attentive walk through a garden, engaging each sense with intention and curiosity.
- By cultivating a deeper awareness of our five senses, we can infuse our lives with greater richness, presence, and appreciation. Each sense offers a unique pathway into the present moment, inviting us to savor the beauty and complexity of our experience. Through regular practice and intention, we can develop a more intimate and joyful relationship with ourselves and the world around us, one sensory experience at a time.

"Talk to yourself like you would to someone you love."

- BRENÉ BROWN

18.
Sound

Your voice is your main superpower! The vibration of your voice can be used to create resonance both internally and externally. Humans have known this for a long time. Many on a spiritual path use their voice to meditate. They may make a repetitive sound such as 'Ommmm…' or chant words repetitively or even recite prayers. This can powerfully shift the nervous system.

It is this vibration, along with the breath, that makes your voice such a unique superpower. The path of the vagus nerve runs very close to our ear. This makes sound a very powerful realm to explore. We are incredibly sensitive to frequencies of sound. For example, you can completely change the meaning of a spoken word by altering the intonation. For example, the word 'No.' It can be used as a complete sentence. The intonation, however, can really change the meaning: 1. No permission given 2. No, that's unbelievable 3. No, I do not. 4. No, thank you, and 5. A question No? All of those different meanings can be inferred, depending on intonation.

The sound of someone's voice can greatly impact how we feel. Hearing the voice of someone you're afraid of can make you feel anxious, even if they're not near you. But hearing the voice of someone you care about can instantly make you feel calm and safe. Our brains are wired this way because we have always listened for signs of danger or safety.

It's really fun to explore all the different notes, rhythms, and textures you can produce just by exhaling while using your voice. Whether you rap an epic melody or beatbox a thumping backbeat, it comes from within you. That's the ultimate instrument you'll ever need!

Another really awesome thing about using your voice and breath for singing, humming, or playing a wind instrument is that it gives you this huge rush of creative power. When you realize you can fill a room with harmonies just by shaping sounds from your vocal cords, it makes you feel like anything is possible!

And the best part is this ability is free and always available to you. It takes courage to open your mouth and let those vocal cords vibrate proudly. Embrace those inner rockstar vibes and show the world the creative magic hiding within your breath!

To reiterate, the main point to remember is that when you interocept safety, you are operating within one branch of your nervous system. *When you get activated due to danger, you leave that branch and operate from a completely different branch of nerves*. It's almost like you are different people in those two states. You may see this in yourself or also in others. This can give you compassion toward others and toward yourself. This is why it is important to clarify your response to the question, "Who am I when I feel safe?" And "Who am I when I feel threatened?" in your own mind.

Bee Yoga Innercise

Place your thumbs in your ears to block sound while covering your eyes with your fingers, blocking your vision.

With a nice long inhale, slowly exhale while making the sound of a bee: "zzzzzzzzzzzzzzzzzzzzzzzzz…"

This is one of my favorites. Bee yoga is an ancient practice. It can actually vibrate the pineal gland or 3rd eye. You may notice a feeling of your skull beginning to vibrate. You may even feel the vibration shift from the left to the right hemisphere. When you stop, what do you notice? Maybe a sense of expansion within the skull?

So, again the ability to focus that vibration and move it around within the body like a Light saber can become like a superpower. You may not realize this until you consciously decide to experiment and explore. The more you use it, the more powerful it gets!

Ear Massage Innercise

Since the vagus nerve runs so close to the ear, it is also possible to shift the nervous system by giving yourself an ear massage. Try it, and you might just like this one;

> Ear Massage
>
> *With your index finger and thumb gently squeezing your earlobe, pull downward.*
>
> *Now pull from the middle area, and pull gently toward the back.*
>
> *At the top of your ear, pull upward.*
>
> *Place your index finger into the ear lobe and make circles forward and backward in the indented area; now do the same above at the top part of the ear.*
>
> *Now place your index finger into your ear canal entry area and gently push forward, upward, backward, and down several times, both ears simultaneously.*
>
> *Pause and note any changes.*

Visual Reset

Lay on your back with your nose pointing to the ceiling.

Without moving your head, move your eyes all the way to the left for 30 seconds.

Release and move your eyes all the way to the right for 30 seconds.

Come back to the center and describe what you notice.

Through the lens of mindful sight, the world reveals itself anew, inviting us to marvel at the extraordinary beauty hidden in the ordinary moments of life.

19.
Sight

Sight is one of our most powerful and dominant senses, playing a crucial role in how we perceive and interact with the world around us. Our eyes allow us to take in vast amounts of information, from the vibrant colors of a sunset to the intricate details of a loved one's face. By learning to harness the power of sight through mindful practices, we can cultivate a deeper sense of presence, gratitude, and connection to the visual wonders that surround us.

Our eyes work by taking in light and converting it into electrical signals that our brain interprets as images. This complex process involves the coordination of many different parts of the eye, including the cornea, lens, retina, and optic nerve. The retina contains millions of light-sensitive cells called rods and cones, which help us distinguish different colors, shapes, and levels of brightness.

The Benefits of Mindful Seeing:

- **Increased Appreciation and Gratitude:** By intentionally focusing on the visual beauty around us, we can cultivate a deeper sense of appreciation and gratitude for the world we live in. This can help shift our perspective towards the positive and improve our overall well-being and happiness.

- **Enhanced Creativity and Problem-Solving**: Engaging in mindful vision practices can stimulate our imagination and creativity, as we learn to look at the world in new and innovative ways. This can also enhance our problem-solving skills, as we become more attuned to visual details and patterns that we might have previously overlooked.

- **Improved Focus and Concentration:** By training our minds to focus on visual stimuli, we can improve our overall ability to concentrate and pay attention. This can be particularly beneficial in today's fast-paced and distraction-filled world, where it can be challenging to stay focused and present.

- **Greater Connection and Empathy:** Mindful seeing can help us develop a greater sense of connection and empathy with others, as we learn to really look at and appreciate the unique qualities and experiences of those around us. This can foster deeper and more meaningful relationships, and contribute to a greater sense of community and understanding.

Incorporating mindful seeing practices into our daily lives can have a profound impact on our overall well-being and perception of the world around us. By learning to see with fresh eyes and an open heart, we can unlock the full potential of this powerful sense, and discover new layers of beauty, meaning, and connection in our everyday experiences. So the next time you open your eyes, remember to really look, and allow yourself to be amazed by the visual wonders that surround you.

Touch is the language of the heart, a gentle reminder of our shared humanity and the healing power of connection.

20.
Touch

Touch is another amazing realm of healing. The frequency of energy radiating outward from your hands can become a superpower. Rub your hands together for a minute. Now face your palms toward one another and sense into feeling a pulsation, like a magnet pulling your hands toward each other and pushing them away from one another. Can you feel into that? This is a ball of your energy that exists at a healing frequency. Now, place your hands around a glass of water and use your intention to infuse that water with a healing frequency. Water carries frequencies, and it carries Light. We can use that wisdom to restore healing frequencies to the body. Remember, your attention and intention are key.

Touch has the power to help restore a sense of safety within. Often, you will feel more settled merely by reaffirming your boundaries to your nervous system.

Touch is a fundamental human need, a sense that connects us to the world around us and to each other in profound and meaningful ways. From the comforting embrace of a loved one to the soothing sensation of a warm bath, touch has the power to heal, nurture, and transform our physical, emotional, and spiritual well-being.

Our skin is the largest organ in the body, containing millions of receptors that respond to various forms of touch, including pressure, temperature, and texture. When we experience positive, nurturing touch, our bodies release oxytocin, a hormone that promotes feelings of bonding, trust, and relaxation. This "cuddle hormone" has been shown to reduce stress, lower blood pressure, and boost immune function, highlighting the vital role that touch plays in our overall health and well-being.

1. Check through the neural vocabulary lists you used in the first Innercise practice to get an idea of your current neural state.
2. Place your right hand under your left armpit and then place your left hand over your right arm.
3. Just pause and take a few breaths - up to about 3 minutes, depending on your current state.
4. What do you feel? What do you notice?
5. Check through the lists again to notice what, if anything, shifted.

The Benefits of Mindful Touch:

- **Stress Reduction and Relaxation:** Engaging in mindful touch practices can help activate the body's relaxation response, reducing stress, anxiety, and tension. By bringing our attention to the present moment and the sensations of touch, we can quiet the mind and find a sense of peace and calm amidst the chaos of daily life.

- **Enhanced Body Awareness and Self-Care:** Mindful touch can help us develop a deeper sense of body awareness, attuning us to the needs and messages of our physical selves. By learning to listen to and respond to these cues with loving, nurturing touch, we can cultivate a greater sense of self-care and compassion, treating ourselves with the kindness and gentleness we deserve.

- **Deeper Connections and Empathy:** Mindful touch can foster deeper, more meaningful connections with others, as we learn to communicate through the language of physical contact. By bringing our full presence and attention to the experience of touching and being touched, we can cultivate greater empathy, understanding, and intimacy in our relationships, both platonic and romantic.

- **Improved Physical Health and Well-being:** Regular, nurturing touch has been shown to have numerous physical health benefits, including boosting immune function, lowering blood pressure, and reducing chronic pain. By incorporating mindful touch practices into our daily lives, we can support our body's natural healing processes and promote overall physical well-being.

Touch is a powerful tool for healing, connection, and transformation, one that we can harness through the practice of mindful awareness. By bringing our full presence and attention to the experience of touch, we can tap into the profound wisdom and nurturing energy of this vital sense, cultivating greater peace, joy, and well-being in all aspects of our lives. So go ahead, reach out and touch the world around you with an open heart and a curious mind, and discover the transformative power of this essential human experience.

Mindful Touch Practices:

- **Self-Massage:** Take a few minutes each day to offer yourself the gift of nurturing touch through self-massage. Use your hands to gently knead and rub your face, neck, shoulders, arms, and legs, paying attention to any areas of tension or discomfort. Use slow, circular motions and experiment with different levels of pressure, noticing how your body responds and relaxes under your own caring touch.
- **Mindful Hugging:** When embracing a loved one, bring your full attention to the experience of touch and connection. Notice the warmth and pressure of the hug, the rhythm of your breathing, and the feelings of love and appreciation that arise. Allow yourself to be fully

present in the moment, savoring the comfort and joy of this simple yet profound act of touch.

- **Texture Exploration:** Gather a variety of objects with different textures, such as a soft feather, a rough stone, a smooth shell, and a fuzzy piece of fabric. Take your time exploring each object with your hands, noticing the subtle sensations and qualities of each texture. Allow yourself to be curious and present, discovering the unique character and beauty of each object through the power of touch.

- **Barefoot Walking:** Find a safe, natural space where you can walk barefoot, such as a sandy beach, a grassy field, or a mossy forest floor. As you walk, bring your attention to the sensations of the earth beneath your feet, noticing the temperature, texture, and contours of the ground. Allow yourself to feel grounded and connected to the earth, drawing strength and nourishment from this primal contact with nature.

"Smell is a potent brain stimulant, capable of enhancing cognitive function, mood & memory"

- RACHEL HERZ

21.
Smell

The Power of Smell: How It Affects Your Nervous System and Well-being

Have you ever wondered how your sense of smell can impact your mood and overall well-being? As one of our five senses, smell plays a significant role in regulating our nervous system and helping us manage stress.

Our sense of smell is directly connected to the part of our brain that processes emotions, memories, and behaviors. This connection allows certain scents to trigger emotional responses and evoke memories, which can greatly influence our mood.

Aromatherapy is a popular practice that harnesses the power of scent to promote relaxation and reduce stress. By using essential oils or scented candles with calming fragrances like lavender, vanilla, or chamomile, you can help your nervous system unwind and find balance.

Pleasant smells can also help lower cortisol levels, the primary stress hormone in the body. When you encounter a soothing scent, it can signal your body to relax and reduce stress, allowing your nervous system to self-regulate more effectively.

In addition to its emotional benefits, your sense of smell plays a vital role in appetite and digestion. The aroma of food can stimulate the production of saliva and digestive enzymes, preparing your body for nourishment.

Certain scents, such as peppermint and citrus, have been shown to improve alertness, concentration, and mental clarity. By incorporating these scents into your environment, you may find it easier to stay focused and productive.

Lastly, the simple act of taking a deep breath and inhaling a pleasant scent can promote relaxation and stress relief. Deep breathing activates the parasympathetic nervous system, which helps calm the body and mind.

By understanding the powerful influence of smell on your nervous system, you can use this knowledge to promote self-regulation and enhance your overall well-being. Try incorporating pleasant scents into your daily life, exploring aromatherapy, and taking moments to appreciate the good smells around you. Your nervous system will thank you for it!

Taste is a sensory gateway to the nervous system, shaping our perceptions, emotions, and physiological responses.

22.
Taste

Taste is one of the five senses that plays a big role in our everyday lives. It not only helps us enjoy different flavors but also influences our mood, memories, and overall health.

When we eat, our tongue and mouth send signals to the brain about the taste of the food. This connection between taste and the brain is why certain foods can make us feel specific emotions or remind us of past experiences.

Comfort foods, like a warm bowl of soup or a slice of homemade pie, often make us feel good. This is because the taste and smell of these foods can cause the brain to release "feel-good" chemicals like serotonin and dopamine.

On the other hand, bitter or sour tastes can sometimes make us feel bad. This is thought to be a built-in response to help us avoid eating foods that might be poisonous or spoiled. However, some people learn to like these tastes over time.

Taste also plays a part in controlling our appetite and eating habits. When we eat something yummy, our brain's reward system is activated, making us want to keep eating. This can be a problem with sugary or fatty foods, as eating too much can lead to health problems.

Mindful eating involves paying close attention to the experience of eating, engaging all of your senses, and being fully present in the moment.

- **Choose a food:** Select a small portion of a food you enjoy, such as a piece of fruit, a bite-sized snack, or a single raisin.
- **Engage your senses:** Before eating, take a moment to observe the food using all of your senses. Look at its colors, shapes, and textures. Notice any aromas. Feel its weight in your hand or on your fork.
- **Slow down:** When you're ready to eat, take a small bite and chew slowly. Focus on the sensations in your mouth, such as the food's texture, temperature, and flavors.
- **Savor the experience:** As you chew, pay attention to how the taste and texture change over time. Notice any thoughts or emotions that arise, but try to let them pass without judgment, returning your focus to the sensations of eating.
- **Check-in with your body:** As you continue eating, periodically pause to check in with your body. Notice any feelings of hunger, fullness, or satisfaction. Ask

yourself if you're enjoying the food and if you want to continue eating.
- **Practice gratitude:** Before finishing your mindful eating exercise, take a moment to reflect on the experience and appreciate the nourishment and enjoyment the food has provided.

By incorporating mindful eating into your daily routine, you can develop a greater appreciation for your food, improve your relationship with eating, and cultivate a more mindful approach to life in general. Remember, mindful eating is a practice, and it may take time to develop this skill. Be patient with yourself and try to approach the experience with curiosity and openness.

Mindful eating is a way to be more aware of how foods taste and to develop a better relationship with what we eat. By enjoying each bite, paying attention to the flavors, and noticing how our body feels, we can make better choices about the foods we eat.

Taste not only affects our mood but also helps our body regulate various functions. For example, the taste of food can make us produce more saliva and digestive enzymes, which helps our body process and use the nutrients from what we eat.

By understanding how important taste is in our lives, we can use it to improve our emotional well-being and make smarter choices about the foods we eat. So, next time you have a meal, take a moment to really taste and enjoy the flavors and remember that taste is not just about the experience but also about taking care of your mind and body.

Innercises can help regulate the nervous system and promote relaxation.

23.
More Innercises

Tune into Your Senses

> - *Drink your favorite hot tea mindfully.*
> - *Notice the warmth, aroma, flavor, and how you feel.*

Our senses can provide clues about what your mind and body need in each moment. Try these sensory practices:

> - *Take a 10-minute technology break.*
> - *No screens, no phones. What do you notice? What sights, sounds, smells, tastes, and textures can you find more easily without those distractions?*
> - *Take a mindful shower or bath - feel the water, listen to sounds, smell soaps, and fully experience.*

Move Your Body and Breathe

Physical movement and focused breathing help reduce anxiety.

- Take a brisk 10-minute walk outside while focusing on the sensations of walking.
- Shake it out - shake your hands, feet, and body loosely while breathing deeply for 30 seconds to reduce tension.
- Try yoga flows such as Sun Salutations to connect movement with breath consciously.

Foster Connection

Supportive relationships boost your mental health.
You could:

- Have an open conversation about how you're feeling with someone you trust.
- Offer sincere compliments to brighten someone's day.
- Spend quality time with a friend or family member doing an activity you both enjoy.
- Volunteer in your community - helping others reduces stress.

Get Proper Rest

Adequate sleep and relaxation boosts mood and focus. Try to:

- *Go to bed and wake up at consistent times to establish a sleep routine.*
- *Power down all screens at least one hour before bedtime.*
- *Try calming activities before bed, like reading, gentle yoga, or drinking herbal tea.*
- *Use a lavender pillow mist or play white noise to create a relaxing sleep environment.*

Take 10-20 minute power naps during the day if you feel a need to recharge.

Tap Into Creativity

Expressing yourself creatively reduces anxiety. Some ideas:

- *Start a daily journal or diary to write your thoughts and feelings.*
- *Make art, poems, music, or photo collages to depict emotions.*
- *Take up hobbies like playing an instrument, knitting, sketching.*
- *Join a school play to act and get into character roles.*
- *Share your creative works with supportive friends and family.*

Foster Self-Confidence

Believing in yourself empowers you to handle challenges. You can:

- List your positive qualities, strengths, skills, and values. Reread it when you feel down.
- Set small attainable goals and celebrate each one you complete.
- Listen to motivating talks or podcasts about self-esteem and the growth mindset.
- Cut yourself some slack - talk to yourself like you would a good friend.

Seek Support If Needed

It's brave to ask for help managing mental health challenges. Consider:

- Talking to a trusted teacher, counselor, or parent about your concerns.
- Joining a peer support group with others facing similar struggles.
- Seeing a therapist or counselor to gain coping skills and process emotions.
- Calling a crisis line if you need immediate support.

Keep Exploring Self-Care

Caring for your mental health is an ongoing, lifelong process.

- *Check in regularly to see what self-care practices work for you as your needs evolve.*
- *Make self-care a priority - your mental health matters!*
- *Learn new tools to care for your mind, body, emotions, creativity, and spirit.*
- *Reach out for help when needed - you don't have to navigate alone.*

"When the nervous system identifies safety, physiology promotes health growth and restoration."

- STEPHEN PORGES

Conclusion

As we come to the end of this journey together, remember that you are never alone. You are an important part of this grand, connected Universe. Your personal experiences, though they may seem individual, also support the whole of humanity and echo throughout the Universe.

Your purpose is both personal and universal. You are a messenger of wisdom and a force for positive change. By embodying love, kindness, and self-care through the daily practice of INNERCISES, you help uplift the collective vibration, contributing to the awakening and evolution of all of humanity.

Every story you share, every insight you gain, has the power to guide others on their own path of self-discovery and healing. Embrace your unique gifts and perspectives, for these are beacons illuminating the way for those who may be struggling. Radiate!

Remember the infinite power that resides within you. Recognize the interconnectedness of all existence, and know that your divine purpose guides your path. You have the ability to master your human experience by awakening the strength, power, and wisdom that lies dormant within through the practice of daily Innercises.

Like a musical symphony, the Universe harmonizes free will, interlocking energies, and infinite possibilities. You are both the creator and the created, the dreamer and the dream. Your intricate blueprint is designed for this higher calling: cultivating inner peace, nurturing your well-being, and radiating your light into the world.

Together, this multidisciplinary approach and the practice of somatic Innercises are your gateways to self-discovery and inner power. They are tools to nourish your spirit and unlock the vast knowledge within the stillness of your own being. Make time for daily practices, meditation, reflection, and self-care practices that resonate with you. In the clarity of your own connection, you will find the next steps on your journey illuminated.

The time is now to embrace your power, to live with the knowingness that you are surrounded by unconditional love and support, guiding you as you navigate this transformative journey of growth and healing.

Remember, you are the key to your well-being and to the collective awakening. Through your courage, self-compassion, and commitment to personal growth, you help birth a new era of unity, understanding, and wholeness. Every step you take, every breath you breathe, every Innercise you practice moves us all toward a new horizon of inner peace and greater power.

So, keep shining your light, keep sharing your stories, and keep nurturing your own well-being. Together, we can build a world where no-cost mental health self-care practices are celebrated and embraced as a path to wholeness and where everyone is empowered to become the best version of their best self.

Glossary

Activation: Feeling really worked up and hyped up, both physically and emotionally, as a reaction to scary stuff or triggers.

Appeasement: Trying to calm down someone or something that seems threatening by being really nice and giving them what they want.

Autonomic Nervous System (ANS): The part of your nervous system that controls automatic body functions like breathing, heart rate, digestion, etc., without you having to think about it.

Befriend: A brain state where you want to connect with others and get their support when things get stressful or dangerous.

Boundaries: Personal limits and rules you set to protect your physical, emotional, and mental space from being invaded.

Coherence: When your body and mind are totally in sync and harmonized.

Collapse: A brain state where you completely shut down physically and mentally, like you're paralyzed and can't function at all.

Co-regulation: How two or more people influence and help regulate each other's physical and emotional states through interactions.

Discharge: Letting out all the built-up energy and tension stored in your body from a really traumatic event so your nervous system can finally chill out and return to normal.

Dysregulation: Basically, when you can't seem to get your physical or emotional states under control.

Embodiment: Integrating your bodily sensations, emotions, and thoughts as one whole experience.

Emotional Regulation: The ability to recognize, understand, and effectively process your emotions to stay balanced and relate to others.

Experiential Anatomy: Learning about your body's anatomy through your own personal experiences and awareness of physical sensations.

Fawning: Trying to people-please and be super agreeable to feel safe and avoid threats.

Felt Sense: A full-body feeling that gives you an intuitive, gut-level understanding of your internal sensations and emotions.

Fight: A brain state where you instinctively want to confront and battle whatever threatens you.

Fight-or-Flight Response: Your body and mind's automatic reaction to danger, controlled by your sympathetic nervous system, prepares you to fight or run away.

Flight: A brain state where you instinctively want to get away and escape from whatever threat you're facing.

Freeze: A brain state where you become so overwhelmed that you are paralyzed and unresponsive when facing a threat to your life, as a way to protect yourself.

Freeze Response: When you freeze up, shut down, and disconnect as a survival strategy to stay safe.

Grounding: Techniques that help you stay present, connected to your body, and aware of your physical environment to feel stable and safe.

Interoception: Your ability to feel and understand the sensations happening inside your body, like emotions, gut feelings, and other physical processes.

Mindfulness: The practice of paying close, non-judgmental attention to the present moment and being aware of your thoughts, sensations, and emotions as they are.

Mobilization: A brain state where your body and mind get super hyped up, alert, and ready for action in response to a threat.

Neural: Anything related to your nervous system or brain cells.

Neuroception: Your brain's unconscious ability to detect whether a situation is safe, dangerous, or socially engaging based on the cues it picks up.

Orienting: Bringing your attention to the present moment and your environment to feel safe and grounded.

Pendulation: The natural swinging back and forth between feeling hyped up and then relaxed as your nervous system heals.

Polyvagal Theory: A theory by Dr. Stephen Porges explaining how your autonomic nervous system controls your social behavior and emotional states.

Posture: How your body is aligned, including your bones, muscles, and overall balance.

Regulation: The ability to get your physical and emotional states under control.

Relational Trauma: Trauma that comes from bad experiences in relationships, often repeated or long-lasting negative stuff with people close to you.

Resilience: Being able to adapt, cope, and bounce back from really tough or traumatic experiences while still feeling good about yourself.

Rest and Digest: A brain state where your body totally relaxes and focuses on restoring itself, controlled by your parasympathetic nervous system.

Resourcing: Building inner strengths and outer support systems to help you regulate yourself and feel safe when dealing with trauma.

Self-Compassion: Treating yourself with kindness, understanding, and acceptance, especially when you're going through a really hard time.

Self-Regulation: The ability to manage and control your inner states, emotions, and behaviors to stay balanced and feel good.

Somatic: Anything related to your physical body and bodily sensations.

Somatic Awareness: Being consciously aware of the sensations in your body, how you move, and your overall felt experiences.

Somatic Experiencing: A type of therapy that focuses on your physical and sensory experiences to help you heal from trauma.

Somatic Intelligence: Your ability to use your bodily sensations, emotions, and gut instincts to make decisions, solve problems, and grow as a person.

Somatic Resilience: Your body and nervous system's ability to adapt, recover, and get back in balance after going through stress, trauma, or dysregulation.

States of Neural Defense: Different ways your nervous system reacts to protect you from perceived threats or danger.

Symbolic Expression: Using non-verbal stuff like art, movement, or writing to express and process your emotions, experiences, and inner states.

Sympathetic Nervous System: The part of your nervous system that activates the "fight-or-flight" response.

Titration: Slowly and carefully explore your traumatic experiences at a pace that allows your nervous system to process them without getting overwhelmed.

Touch and Bodywork: Therapies that involve physically touching the body, like massage or acupuncture, to support healing and regulation.

Tracking: Paying attention to the sensations, movements, and changes happening in your body to increase self-awareness and regulation.

Trauma: Super difficult and overwhelming experiences that are too much for you to handle, often messing up your nervous system's regulation and causing ongoing issues.

Trauma Vortex: A state of dysregulation where traumatic memories and sensations become so intense and overwhelming that they're really hard to process.

Vagus Nerve: The longest nerve in your body that plays a huge role in controlling many bodily functions. It activates all systems at once out of safety to states of neural defense (fight, flight, freeze)

Window of Tolerance: The ideal range of physical and emotional activation levels where you can effectively deal with stress and engage in healthy behaviors.

	My thoughts	I feel	My body is...	My actions are
When safe:	Curious Clear mind Creative Flexible Focus and concentration Positive outlook	Happy Joy Love Even mood Grateful Confident Comfortable	Vibrant Relaxed muscles Even breath Moderate heart rate Easy digestion elimination Expressive facial movements Vocal prosody	Attuned Responsive Interactive Patient Trusting
Fight Or Flight:	Over/ or unfocused Difficult concentration Negative outlook Rigid Repetitive thoughts Rapid thoughts	Irritable Grumpy Annoyed Spiteful Angry Rage Worried Anxious Afraid Terror Panic	Tight muscles Fast, shallow breath Fast heart rate Cold hands&feet Sweaty and hot Dry mouth Poor digestion Constipation Restless Agitated Shaky Fast speech Eyes darting Poor sleep	Impatient Self-focused Confrontational Avoidant Defensive Offended
Freeze:	Hopeless Stuck Trapped Frozen Scattered Spacey Dreamy Confusion Blank mind Forgetful	Numb Apathy Shame Paralyzed Shocked	Very tight or overly soft muscles Slow heart rate Slow, shallow breathing Numbness Dizziness Pale Blurry vision Flat facial expression Monotone voice Clumsy	Disconnected Non-responsive Shut down Checked out Isolated

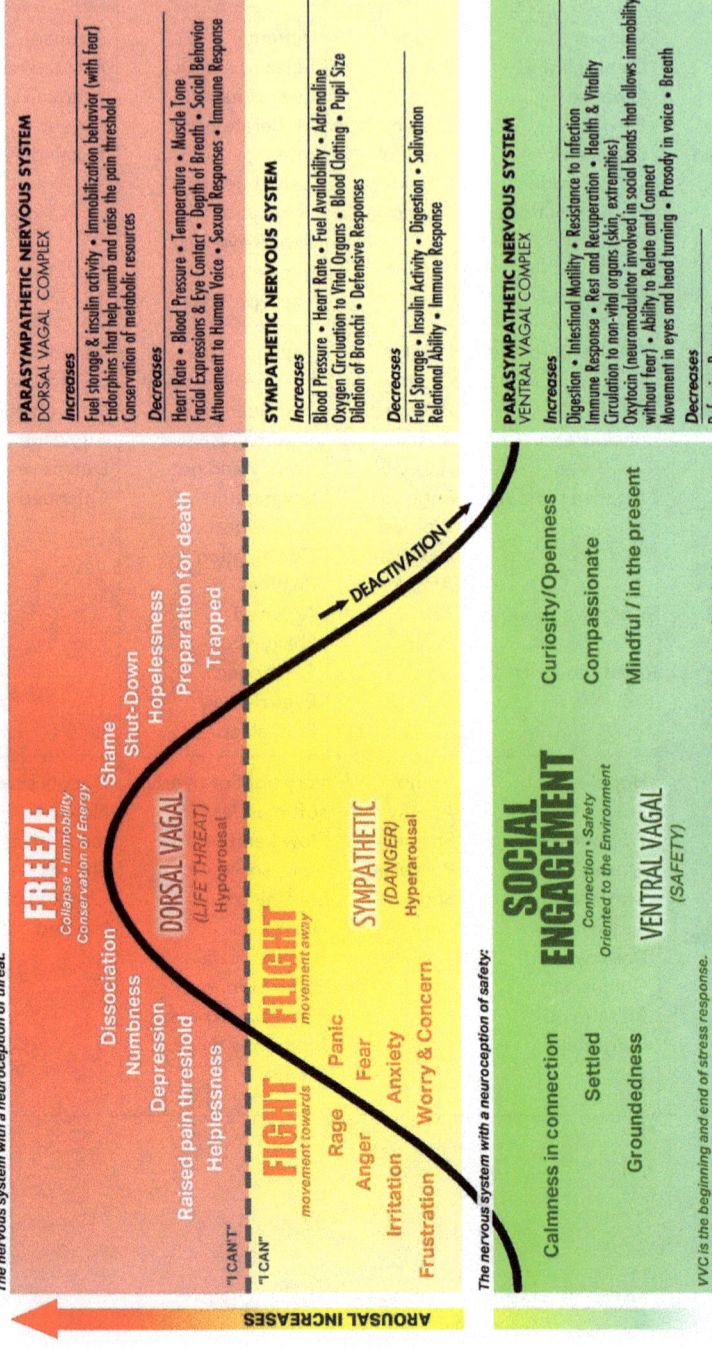

www.ingramcontent.com/pod-product-compliance
Lightning Source LLC
Chambersburg PA
CBHW060524030426
42337CB00015B/1988